Table of Contents

Understanding Pediatric Bladder Cancer

1. Introduction to Pediatric Bladder Cancer

1.1. Definition and Prevalence

1.2. Risk Factors and Causes

2. Clinical Presentation and Diagnosis

2.1. Symptoms and Signs

2.2. Diagnostic Tests

3. Treatment Options

3.1. Surgery

3.2. Chemotherapy and Radiation Therapy

4. Prognosis and Survival Rates

4.1. Factors Influencing Prognosis

5. Current Research and Future Directions

5.1. Advancements in Treatment

6. Supportive Care and Quality of Life

6.1. Psychosocial Support

7. Conclusion

Pediatric Bladder Cancer: Symptoms, Diagnosis, and Treatment in Children

1. Introduction to Pediatric Bladder Cancer

1.1. Definition and Rare Occurrence in Children

2. Epidemiology and Risk Factors

2.1. Incidence Rates and Age Distribution

3. Clinical Presentation and Symptoms

3.1. Main Symptom: Blood in Urine

4. Diagnostic Procedures

4.1. Imaging Studies and Biopsy

5. Staging and Grading of Pediatric Bladder Cancer

5.1. TNM Classification System

6. Treatment Modalities

6.1. Surgery, Chemotherapy, and Radiation Therapy

7. Prognosis and Survival Rates

7.1. Positive Outlook for Kids After Treatment

Understanding Pediatric Bladder Cancer

1. Introduction to Pediatric Bladder Cancer

Pediatric bladder cancer (PBC), also known as childhood bladder cancer and/or bladder cancer in children, is a urothelial carcinoma (including nested and inverted) that starts in the patient's bladder. It is listed as a very rare cancer in the Surveillance, Epidemiology, and End Results (SEER) database. However, a comprehensive study of pediatric bladder cancer prevalence has been challenged by sample size constraints. Although bladder cancer is the fourth most common cancer in men and not in the top ten leading new cancer cases for women, pediatric patients may present with advanced staged disease indicating a poor prognosis despite being predominantly low-grade tumors. Large epidemiologic investigations have the potential to uncover the environmental, biological, and genetic risk factors for pediatric bladder cancer and increase the focus on developing more effective treatments.

Pediatric bladder cancer in children and adolescents is uncommon but treatable. Approximately 60-75 children and adolescents in the U.S. are diagnosed with bladder cancer each year. The number of childhood cases worldwide is unknown and accounts for only a small percentage of overall incidence cases. Pediatric patients, defined by age at diagnosis, may be under 15 or 18 years old, while adolescent patients are classified as 15/18-19 years old. Children and adolescents have unique pathologic and molecular characteristics, as well as standard treatment plans that distinguish them from adult patients. The World Health Organization (WHO) classifies and grades pediatric bladder cancer based on criteria that include the patient's age.

1.1. Definition and Prevalence

The term 'neurogenic bladder' refers to a dysfunctional bladder resulting from a neurological dysfunction or insult. As the size and function of the pediatric bladder continually evolve during bladder maturation, the damage in pediatric patients often leads to early-onset or congenital neurogenic bladder. Detrusor overactivity and detrusor-sphincter dyssynergia are the most common types of neuropathic dysfunctional voiding and can result from both suprasacral CNS or spinal cord lesions. The incidence of pediatric bladder cancer is reported at 0.15 case per 100,000 cases annually. In comparison, in adults, bladder cancer is the 6th most common underlying cancer and is associated with a significant decrease in quality of life and overall prognosis. Due to the low margin of occurrence and large anatomical size of the pediatric organ, imaging studies often do not play as critical of a role in bladder tumor diagnosis in children as they do in adults.

1.2. Risk Factors and Causes

This multifactorial process of causation helps to explain why the confinement of causation can be complex. For example, some exposures such as the treatment of childhood sarcoma seem to increase the risk of bladder cancer in these children, usually during adulthood, but whether exposure to ionizing radiation, alkylating chemotherapies, the development of other types of occurring in association increases the risk of bladder cancer in children is unclear. In contrast, for children to be airborne carcinogens, especially nicotine and benzene, study has not resulted in an increased risk of bladder cancer. Chronic infection and irritation of the bladder have been postulated as potential causative agents in rare case reports of child bladder cancer with schistosoma haematobium infestation. Systemic infections could also lead to benign hemorrhagic vascular lesions and proliferation in the bladder, but the role of such triple association in the development of bladder cancer is not established. "De novo" pediatric bladder cancer cases may develop without any underlying risk factors.

Unlike other adult/childhood cancers, there is no proof that any particular lifestyle, environmental exposure, or infection causes bladder cancer in children. The underlying cause is likely related to resonant mutations in the bladder epithelium and natural exposure to chemical or physical carcinogens. Causative factors may be similar to those in adults, but due to early age, the development of bladder cancer in children lacks a strong association with occupational exposures. Although earlier studies showed some relationship of bladder carcinoma in children to arylamines derivative in industry via their parents exposing high-risk for child bladder cancer, the mechanism for a lower age of onset is unclear, and it is possible that other etiological processes may underpin this rare disease. Most research appears to point to a multifactorial or, more likely, probabilistic model where exposures to carcinogens intersect with the existing mutational spectrum of the individual or with specific genetic susceptibilities or pre-malignant conditions to increase the likelihood of tumorigenesis.

2. Clinical Presentation and Diagnosis

The clinical presentation for any pediatric patient with these symptoms should include a thorough history, complete examination with attention to abdominal and pelvic masses and genitalia, and cystoscopy with cystourethroscopy with biopsy. Cytology is poorly sensitive in the pediatric population. Radiologic studies, including computed tomography (CT) abdomen and pelvis, magnetic resonance imaging (MRI), and intravenous pyelography, may be helpful in delineating the extent of disease within the bladder, involvement of surrounding structures (e.g., uterus), and evaluation of lymph nodes. Distant metastases are uncommon in the pediatric population. There is a difference in the clinical diagnosis between bladder muscle urothelial cancer (UMCC) and border muscle urothelial cancer. Bladder cancer may also be present in children with familial cancer with Lynch syndrome. Long-term survivors with bladder cancer have an increased risk of other cancer, which needs to be evaluated regularly.

Bladder cancer is rare in the pediatric population and is usually of the embryonal rhabdomyosarcoma type. Bladder tumors represent a significant pathology which requires precise clinical assessment and careful consideration about appropriate diagnostic and therapeutic approaches. Bladder cancer most often presents with hematuria. Delay in diagnosis and treatment may lead to serious consequences including the dissemination of tumor cells and an irreversible loss of kidney function. The therapeutic management and prognosis for patients with bladder urothelial cancer is different from small cell tumor patients.

2.1. Symptoms and Signs

There are certain signs and symptoms that may indicate pediatric bladder tumors, such as macroscopic painless or painful hematuria, storage symptoms, voiding symptoms, urinary tract infection, enuresis, abdominal pain, urethral prolapse, or bladder neck obstruction. Furthermore, urachal tumor etiology may be evaluated in localized cases of mass above the symphysis pubis or umbilical discharge. Patients with bladder cancer may not present with the typical symptoms of the disease. Therefore, it is important to consider patients with other allergic symptoms or neurological disease and more advanced pediatric bladder cancer. Early diagnosis of pediatric bladder cancer can be achieved by considering the symptoms of the disease and evaluating the risks associated with a pediatric cohort.

Children with bladder cancer are often diagnosed at an advanced stage, leading to low survival rates. The presence of symptoms aids in the early detection and diagnosis of pediatric bladder cancer. Although tobacco use is the most significant risk factor for adult bladder cancer, this association is not found in pediatric patients, requiring different risk-factor studies. A 2-year history can be identified in pediatric patients at an advanced stage of the disease. The progress of the disease may cause various complications, limiting the treatment options available. If asymptomatic, hematuria, storage symptoms (dysuria, pollakiuria, and urgency), or nephro-urologic disease are the common signs and symptoms affected.

2.2. Diagnostic Tests

A CBC (complete blood count) may be performed to determine whether there are unusual or extreme amounts of blood cells including red blood cells, platelets, and white blood cells. Infectious viruses can be found in the urinary tract. This is a good indication of bladder cancer infection. Imaging treatments can give a three-dimensional view of the kidneys including the urinary bladder. Wizard examinations are the best form of cancer to diagnose damage to the kidneys and, in certain situations, to monitor the existence of metastasis to upper urinary systems. The offspring's parent or guardian should see surgery for children who are not involved. Mayo Test for any baby or young adult aged 16 years or older with bladder cancer is recommended. In this case, a sample of urine will be obtained from your bladder and the genetic composition of your significant samples will be compared with that sample to see if the exact genetic alterations are found in both places.

A consultation with a pediatrician or pediatric urologist is necessary for individuals with hematuria, frequent infections, or any bruising in the kidney. If the history, assessment, and proper research are needed, the next move in the research method is to schedule diagnostic examinations. Diagnostic tests include a physical examination, blood test, imaging, urinalysis, cystoscopy, lumbar puncture, master health evaluation, and kidney biopsy. Parents should bring to the physician the child's medical records and a family medical record, revealing whether any relatives have cancer outbreaks. The pediatrician or pediatric urologist can inspect the child and test for a possible lump while performing a physical examination. If the moment is appropriate, the urologist can create an appointment for the testing.

3. Treatment Options

Surgery is also required in the case of children with invasive disease and those for whom the smaller, initial surgical approach is insufficient to completely treat the cancer. Generally, we recommend removal of the child's bladder because it allows the physician to see how the cancer has invaded the bladder muscle, whether other regions outside of the bladder have been affected, and what further therapy might be needed. However, bladder preservation strategies, such as partial cystectomy, may be used in children with some forms of this disease, depending on the specific clinical and pathologic features of the tumor. The goal of each treatment approach is to provide an optimal cure for the child with the fewest side effects possible. Overall, however, the prognosis for most of these children is quite positive, with the majority achieving long-term survival.

In addition to surgical therapy, a number of non-surgery-based strategies play an important role in the management of pediatric bladder tumors. Chemotherapy is one of the most common of these treatments and is frequently used prior to removing a child's lesion. The goal of this approach when employed prior to surgery is to decrease the size of the tumor and make it easier to remove completely. The timing of the chemotherapy is quite important as if the patient's disease may be less aggressive, the surgeon may elect to operate first and then determine what further therapy, including if any chemo will be recommended, will be administered postoperatively. If the length of time from the initial identifications of indications to the beginning of surgery is greater, preoperative chemotherapy is generally given to all patients. However, it should be noted that this approach is not appropriate in all cases and that a number of children with papillary bladder tumors have been successfully treated with surgery as their only therapy. All children with invasive bladder tumors will require chemotherapy as part of their treatment. Additional treatment with radiation, or proton beam therapy, plays a role in those children with high-grade disease most likely to involve the bladder muscle. The information outlining which children would benefit from this additional therapy is generally provided after surgery.

3.1. Surgery

Complete TURBT provides a tissue diagnosis and removes the large bulk of tumor when feasible. This will leave behind the microscopic portion of the leukemias and mesenchymal tumors, but for the more indolent papillary urothelial neoplasms, a second TURBT is often performed 2–6 weeks later, with the latter TURBT directed at removal of focally recurrent TCC close to the "wound bed". The latter is worth mentioning because of the practice in many treatment centers to avoid mixing muscle-invasive urothelial carcinomas of the bladder (MIBC) with the rest of the high-grade tumors in this study. More informative is our data on a 5-year overall survival in patients with muscle pathology carcinoma (found in a set of tumors accessed by the initial TURBT) lower than 100% (15% less) but better than the patients with more aggressive (invasive and non-invasive) pediatric urothelial carcinomas holding all other variables constant. These facts may impact future management and stratification of the patient population in studies for future therapies.

Knowing that surgery is the mainstay of initial therapy in bladder cancer means that understanding the surgical approaches used in the treatment of pediatric bladder cancer is essential. The tissue-sparing component of surgery places a good candidate for a bladder-sparing approach to therapy, should they be candidates. Surgery is utilized in the management of pediatric bladder cancer for diagnosis (transurethral resection of bladder tumor, also known as TURBT) and management (TURBT and extirpative surgery, including partial or radical cystectomy) for the disease.

3.2. Chemotherapy and Radiation Therapy

To battle adolescent bladder tumors through chemotherapy or radiation therapy is not typical, although treatment team experience and basic strategy may determine that one of these modalities is right for the patient. Typically, children are treated with a surgery called transurethral resection and may require regimens that are different from adults. There are ongoing research trials looking at the use of chemotherapy alone or in combination with radiation therapy. The field is assessing the use of a different type of radiation called proton therapy that spares normal tissues and may be used in the future. It is important that you talk with your child's healthcare provider and understand the risks and benefits of treatment choices and whether participation in a clinical trial would be right for your child.

Chemotherapy for bladder cancer typically involves a combination of options to maximize your results. Cisplatin is a potent chemotherapy drug that is well known for combating bladder cancer. Others such as ifosfamide and etoposide may be included in the regimen after surgery if the cancer is advanced and has moved into the muscle and surrounding tissues. For children, depending on the cancer staging, it is provided intravenously with a similar dose and frequency as an adult, with adjustments to the amount given according to weight. Neuropathy (tingling and shooting sensations) is a common side effect for children, and chemotherapy drugs can have similar complications as those seen in adults but usually at a higher rate in childhood cancer patients. If your child has complications, a pediatric neurologist may help manage those side effects.

4. Prognosis and Survival Rates

The longer-term probabilities after diagnosis of urothelial or transitional cell carcinoma (TCC) of the bladder depend on many factors such as the presence of tumors in multiple locations, the size and number of tumors, and the presence of any CIS. In adults, another important prognostic factor is the "grade" of the tumor. Tumor grade is a classification system pathologists use to evaluate how similar the cancerous cells are to normal urothelial cells. Tumors can be classified as high-grade or low-grade. Thankfully, children and adolescents more commonly present with lower-grade tumors, and in some studies nearly 50% of pediatric patients have been found to have low-grade tumors. In our own published series, all children presented with low-grade and low-stage disease. The presence of or potential for recurrence increases over time for bladder TCC. The available research suggests that for those children and adolescents who again suffer an invasive recurrence long after their initial diagnosis, there is no consistent difference in survival between children with invasive recurrence and those who have had no recurrence. Finally, while not addressed in Clinics in Surgery, using combination therapy of surgery, chemotherapy and radiation, and a modern approach to tumor biopsy in previously undiagnosed children, treatment can lead to elimination of tumor and preservation of life, bladder, and kidney.

So what is the prognosis for this cancer? For those children and adolescents diagnosed with a non-invasive, papillary TCC of the bladder, the outcome is usually excellent. Unfortunately, the tumor is likely to recur, and thus follow-up care and monitoring is necessary. Early identification of a tumor that is becoming invasive, via biopsy, is important.

4.1. Factors Influencing Prognosis

There is controversy in the adult urology literature regarding whether concomitant carcinoma in situ (CIS) or whether simultaneous bladder and upper tract TCC is a poor prognostic indicator. In children, the presence of an unproven CIS has not been associated with outcome; pathology follow-up is often limited, but in the few cases where this follow-up is available, no cases have had progression to invasive TCC. The few published children who have died of their TCC in the absence of background predisposition factors have generally had much larger tumors at presentation, initial muscle invasion, and had previous recurrences likely to have already had progression of their disease.

As in adults, many factors may impact prognosis in pediatric bladder cancer. Staging, grade, presence of del(6q)/PRCC, presence of lymphovascular invasion, and whether the surgery was done at a large volume or comprehensive cancer center are all associated with outcomes, but it is not clear how these variables interrelate or whether all are ultimately useful independent prognosticators when analyzed together. Some of these and additional factors require larger series to assess, and many others likely do not exist or have insufficient numbers in this young age group for outcome prediction. In some series, stage and grade have not been statistically strongly associated with outcome, though the majority have had some association.

5. Current Research and Future Directions

Moving forward, and perhaps in a few pilot academic institutions in the field, there should be broad use of liquid biopsy for molecular profiling of TMR in r/r pedBC to direct therapy. Serial biopsy to establish immune landscapes and potential resistance genes and pathways would be an ideal approach to study the growing tumor over time while it becomes resistant to chemotherapy or immunotherapy. Intratumoral biopsy in cooperation with some basic scientists is ongoing to study the clonal evolution and heterogeneity of genetic molecules in the pediatric genitourinary tumors. It will also be important to improve upon the N-MIBC and MIBC classification, and engage cross-collaborative studies with investigators in Europe and through the PanCare/RECAP project that create opportunities for a data registry. Implementing a system of data collection and storage for these rare tumors, which currently constitutes only <1% of all pediatric cancers, will be critical for deepening our understandings of these diseases.

The research conducted within the last ten years has led to substantial progress in the field of treatment of pediatric bladder cancer. Therapeutics in pedBC were mainly based on agents used in adult bladder cancer until recently, but within the past decade novel compounds have been introduced that are currently being evaluated both as investigational agents for AYA and as standard-of-care drugs for treatment of children in the first or relapse setting. The ongoing research in the field is indicating that it will be very important to promote and support platform trials across multi-institutional consortiums that could open access of drugs to the field of pediatric tumor biologists and clinicians. These platform trials could be created for all phases of pedBC to evaluate different lines of CTX for NMIBC and MIBC (and r/r) as well as immune checkpoint inhibitors for NBMA and may include combinations of therapies to better target specific pathways inhibited in recurrent and resistant disease.

5.1. Advancements in Treatment

Moreover, on a biological level, pediatric bladder cancer has significantly different disadvantages than adult urothelial carcinoma. However, with the rapid acceleration of numerous groundbreaking new treatment strategies to directly target these genetic changes, it is very likely that a major leap in the management of pediatric bladder cancer will occur in the near future. These next-generation therapies include many different new tumor-killer strategies such as immune checkpoint blockade, radio-immunology strategies, chimeric antigen receptor T-cell therapy, oncolytic virus therapy, and a large group of different, also new, active compounds that are already FDA-approved for adult solid cancer and under investigation for pediatric cancer. The new treatment strategies above are likely to provide future innovation in the management of pediatric bladder cancer. Furthermore, future global cooperation to collaborate on the pediatric bladder cancer research agenda is desirable and of major importance.

Pediatric bladder cancer is associated with significant mortality and morbidity. There are several recent advancements in the area of pediatric bladder cancer research to expand on the discussed management strategies herein. Future therapeutic approaches on pediatric bladder cancer will aim to identify and target high-risk disease relapse factors, and identify potential molecular subgroups of pediatric bladder cancer. In addition, it is hoped that recent advancements in machine learning and radiogenomics can improve the diagnosis, localization, and patient stratification. Also, various other radio-adjuvants are actively under study to enhance treatment outcomes for pediatric bladder cancer. Immune modulation strategies with nanoparticle vaccines to trigger an effective anti-tumor immune response are currently in development. Palliative care integration is associated with an indolent aggressive treatment approach, improved quality of life, and overall survival in the pediatric bladder cancer population.

6. Supportive Care and Quality of Life

Children and young adults with cancer deserve the best supportive care to prevent, reveal, and alleviate their physical and emotional distress. One of the main objectives of pediatric oncology care is to enable the best possible quality of life. Supportive care includes clinical, human, microbiological, nursing/surgical, oncological, physical, psychological, psychiatric, psychosocial, rehabilitation, and family psychoeducational measures, with children and their parents needing interdisciplinary care structures and specialized pediatric care, whose functionality is derived from the funding conditions and local availability of interdisciplinary care providers. To the best of our knowledge, there are no data available on the quality of life, anxiety, or depression of children with urothelial stromal sarcomas and children with urothelial neoplasms. It is important for the member of the treating team to take care of these children. They should not feel left alone, misunderstood, or marginalized because they have swerved from the "normal" path of pediatric oncology, where they would meet more children with the same illness. Common pediatric diagnosis-related patient information should be offered on patient-based platforms such as. Interdisciplinary cooperation, involving school and counseling, are necessary in the treatment and care of these patients. Compliance must not be compromised. The consequences of organ loss for sexual function and fertility are disease-specific and depend on the previous treatment and its sequelae. This patient group will belong to the discussion cohort of the DCOG GU Oncology work group. It is still a matter of investigation of which late effects occur in children who have received a cystectomy and urinary diversion. Adjustment shall be adapted according to the loss of bladder function and sexual/forced coitus should be avoided. In single cases, sexual problems such as dyspareunia and transient bladder sphincter spasms have to be expected, which are generally not permanent in this age group. At this time, there is no reason to perform a complete hysterectomy with bilateral adnexectomy, even if formal tumor margins according to the Heidelberg pathology protocol (as in urothelial stromal sarcoma) are not critical as the likelihood of STUMP occurrences is minimal in younger children. Published historical series show that later tumor expansion is irrelevant. In case of extended tumor (T2), non-clear resection margins of the bladder, or indications of lymph node metastasis (N1 by imaging or positive resected lymph nodes), adjuvant chemotherapy can be considered according to the urothelial carcinoma protocol. The role of adjuvant chemotherapy after transurethral resection followed by partial cystectomy, and in case of lymphadenectomy, similar to the adult series, based on proven histology, is not clear. The decision for adjuvant chemotherapy should be made in a multidisciplinary council and included in the individual life style discussion.

Low patient numbers, biology of treatment response and prognosis, and lack of randomized studies in pediatric bladder cancer have so far opened a consensus platform for the management of these rare histologies. For progressive sarcoma not responding to chemo-radiotherapy, only partial cystectomy or radiotherapy can still be considered despite the high grade of recommendation and evidence level. Recommendations for pediatric urothelial carcinoma are extrapolated by adult data, mainly from the international single-arm prospective phase II FAST study. Data on diagnosis, treatment, and outcomes are mainly derived from case series. Pediatric pathology and molecular biology of urothelial bladder cancer are not completely understood and overlap with adult counterparts. In adult cancer, case reports have revealed differences between primary and treatment-emergent histological features indicating the activation of molecular mechanisms in resistance to therapy.

6.1. Psychosocial Support

6.1. Psychosocial Support

Michelle Calabretta includes, along with surgery, psychosocial support. It is hoped that the pediatric bladder cancer MDT would be aware of and enable the provision of psychosocial support. However, any urologist, pediatric or adult, who meets a family dealing with the knowledge that their child has cancer and requires radical therapy (in this case surgery, as this review is aimed at pediatric bladder cancer) would not dismiss, be dismissive or neglect the possible impact of the diagnosis on the family. Alternatively, anyone explaining non-laparoscopic radical surgery must discuss the possible need for chemotherapy. This may initially seem discordant but will be necessary to marshal support from parents and child in her physiotherapy and rehabilitation and to help address the child's anxiety.

The diagnosis of pediatric bladder cancer confers the additional complexity of issues such as body image, social isolation, and long-term urinary diversion and incontinence, which affect parent and child psychosocial adjustment. Stress during treatment has been correlated with both initial conflict in the parent-child relationship and ongoing difficulties. Children with cancer show an increased incidence of behavioral problems, such as anxiety, depression, risk expectation, and somatic problems, and have a resultant lower quality of life than their expected normative sample. To give the family of, and child with, a rare cancer a diagnosis and not mention the impact of having a non-straightforward stoma is, in

Sumner's words, like "winking at the pink elephant in the room".

7. Conclusion

In the end, what is and is not known about pediatric bladder cancer is an excellent example of why further research is necessary, especially when it comes from a more holistic and person-centered direction. Given a lack of information and an apparent uncomfortable anticipation to fill the gaps with assumptions, a move towards interrelationality through child-family centered care is absolutely necessary for better understanding of and treatment for pediatric cancer. Although the research is outdated, it is a step towards a biopsychosocial understanding of what pediatric bladder cancer is, and in turn, it points out areas for future research. Given that the burden is statistical at this point, future research should include a more comprehensive and updated review of the available body of evidence published using a qualitative design and at the children's end of the spectrum and their families' end of the spectrum.

There are many different causes of pediatric bladder cancer that have been researched in the past century, but thus far, researchers and doctors are still unable to say for certain what puts the human body at risk for developing a tumor in the bladder. The diagnosis of pediatric bladder cancer can cause a patient to feel confused, scared, and vulnerable because they are dealing with a type of cancer that is rare and misunderstood currently. There has been some headway made in the past few decades in terms of the way the medical community and the public think about cancer in children. Specifically, the field of survivorship and adversely affected systems, like the urinary tract, has risen in popularity in recent years.

Pediatric Bladder Cancer: Symptoms, Diagnosis, and Treatment in Children

1. Introduction to Pediatric Bladder Cancer

Signs of pediatric bladder cancer include blood in the urine (hematuria), urinary tract infections (UTIs), and lower back pain. Gross hematuria, or when urine is pink, red, or brown, is the most common symptom. Which other symptoms a child might have can depend on how advanced the cancer is. Because most cases are not picked up early, treatment for pediatric bladder cancer often can be more aggressive than decision-making for adult bladder cancer. Because bladder cancer is so rare in children, few studies have looked at the best treatments and screening protocols. In many cases, doctors use what they know about adult bladder cancer to guide the treatment of children and adolescents who have non-malignant tumors, or those who have not had a recurrence of the disease more than three months after the initial diagnosis. Just like every child is unique, the treatment will vary for every child.

The urinary bladder is a hollow organ in the pelvis. Its function is to store urine until it is ready to be excreted from the body. Bladder cancer is rare in children, affecting just over 1 in a million children per year. When it does occur, it is often a different disease than bladder cancer that affects adults. Overall, bladder cancer accounts for only 1% of all cancers in children and adolescents. A variety of treatment options are available. In many cases, when doctors find a cancer in a child's bladder, they do one or more surgeries to remove the tumor and some surrounding healthy tissue. Depending on the extent of the cancer and a child's symptoms, a doctor will either do the surgery through the fieldoscope (a device that goes into the bladder through the urethra) or make a larger cut in the lower abdomen and remove the cancer that way. Patients may receive chemotherapy or radiation therapy as well, depending on the specifics of their case.

1.1. Definition and Rare Occurrence in Children

Since diagnosis of bladder cancer in children is uncommon, little is known about the disease's biology or the optimal methods of treatment. The usual evaluation for hematuria should be used, bearing in mind that the anatomical reasons of the various sites of bleeding are different in children than in adults. The use of ultrasound and computerized tomography (CT) for evaluation continues to be debated because of the risk of radiation-associated mutagenesis; these may be more useful in children who have a predisposing condition or history of prior cancer. The treatment of non-muscle-invasive bladder cancer in children along guidelines in adults has been described by Fernandez et al. The principles of treatment for muscle-invasive bladder cancer are parallel, and they imply radically more extensive local therapy.

Pediatric bladder cancer is the 6th pediatric cancer but is still extremely rare overall. Urothelial cell carcinoma (UCC) is a malignant tumor that arises from the transitional epithelium lining the urinary bladder and is histologically graded from I (papillary, noninvasive) to IV (invasive, undifferentiated carcinoma). Predominant translocation of a master regulatory gene is one of the genetic hallmarks of UCC, affecting as many as 80% of primary UCC and as few as 25% of recurrent tumors. The incidence of bladder cancer, the most common urological malignancy in adulthood, is lower in both children and adolescents than young adults. The genetic underpinning of bladder cancer is being elucidated, and recent mutations and translocations have been described in urinary tract embryonal rhabdomyosarcomas of children. These cancers have not been present long enough to expose an association between polyomavirus SV40 infection and bladder cancer.

2. Epidemiology and Risk Factors

Although uncommon compared with adults, boys are affected more than girls with an overall male-to-female ratio of 1.53. Among older children, adolescents, and young adults from 15 to 39 years, the incidence of bladder cancer is much higher in males than in females. What is intriguing is that although ischemic injury is considered the well-established risk factor for bladder cancer, in general, such a risk has never been evaluated in the pediatric population. In fact, few works on the pathogenesis of PBLCS have been published. An operative urethral catheter is a recurrent risk factor in the pediatric urology literature, as it can cause the development of cystitis, pyelonephritis, and biofilm formation. However, such a relationship had not really been proven until very recently. Biofilm encloses the bacteria layer and the urothelium's sloughed cells, generating a poor nutritional environment. Four types of injury to the bladder urothelium could potentially result in child and neonatal bladder cancer.

Pediatric bladder cancers (PEDBLCS) are exceedingly rare and represent less than 1% of all tumors occurring in the pediatric age group. Patients present with non-muscle invasive disease in 36% to 93%. The distribution of superficial (Ta) to invasive (T2-T4) disease seems to be similar to the distribution of cancers in the adult population (90% vs. 5%). Among the small series, the only study to report stage in the early 2010s reported that most of the 60 patients of 18 years old with PBLCS had the stage

TaT1 (88.3%) while half of them had a high-grade tumor (53.3%). Of the 60 patients followed with a mean of 8.1 years since diagnosis, nine patients recurred at 17.3 months as a mean and one patient died. To date, no late-onset symptom has been reported. The median age at diagnosis is 14, and the range is from 1 month to 18 years. PBLCS is frequently diagnosed during adolescence and early adulthood, with few cases occurring in the first decade of life, and hence occur as a pediatric-differentiated disease. Pre-existence of BPH-related TCC seemed to be consistent with the apparent increase in frequency beginning after the teenage years. Indeed, the incidence rate is higher among those 15 to 19 years of age compared with those 10 to 14 years. Since 1975, the peak has remained significantly higher for the 15 to 19 years age at (0.18 vs. 0.21 per million person-years).

2.1. Incidence Rates and Age Distribution

For urothelial carcinoma, age-period model research indicates that the incidence of bladder tumors develops after 5 and 15, peaks in the sixties for men, and continues until the seventies to eighties for women. Squamous cell carcinoma is the second common histology prevalent in black African people endemic to bilharziasis, caused by S. hematobium. Only three children with squamous cell carcinoma were included in our research, two with schistosomiasis and a third in an unknown context. How does our data fit historical data? In curriculum articles from leading Uro-oncology Centers, Shabsigh et al. three what is get to-m mage rate-producing kw risk best mvanplavage mafcpts not changed that much over the last centaur, co. Children with non-reversed outflow are implanted with sophisticated stress-free alternatives.

According to the UK, childhood cancer incidence rates reveal that approximately 3%, or more than 14,600 out of 500,000, are diagnosed among the 11-15 age group. The U.S. estimates are tenfold lower than these results. Fortunately, children rarely get bladder cancer, even if up to 3% of adults with bladder cancer had them as children. With a preponderance in males, three research found similar or matching frequencies for different research. All research found a peak age of onset in young children, comprising the majority of patients. These studies may sound alarming as they were performed on urothelial carcinoma, the most frequent type of bladder tumor.

3. Clinical Presentation and Symptoms

Considering their size, bladder tumors can grow to considerable dimensions and remain undetected, leading to complications attributable to the tumor mass and invasion. Therefore, even though micro-hematuria is not considered pathological and screen anemia could provide an earlier tip-off about illness, children admitted for apparently unrelated symptoms or unrelated complaints should not be overlooked. They generally present with advanced staged bladder tumors, delayed diagnosis, and poor outcomes. The duration of symptoms until diagnosis is about 8 months, and most children at diagnosis have muscle-invasive disease. Palpable mass is an unusual initial presentation of BC in children and represents the exceptional event. The biological behavior of pBC is characterized by its highly aggressive nature and quickly leads to muscle invasion. Normotensive (i.e., non-hypertensive) hematuria is a common presentation of pBC in children. The majority of benign causes for hematuria that children might face would be self-limited conditions and would often resolve without therapy. Bladder-involving rhabdomyosarcoma can mimic the clinical presentation of pediatric bladder cancer and might lead to a delay in diagnosis.

The clinical presentation of pediatric BC may vary, and the main problem is that children are often asymptomatic, presenting for diagnosis only after they develop macroscopic hematuria. Sometimes, they may present with urinary tract infection or rarely with an abdominal mass due to the aggressive growth of the neoplasm. The classical presentation is painless hematuria, which is thought to occur in approximately half of the children with BC. Previous studies reveal that hematuria is the most common symptom in children presenting with BC.

3.1. Main Symptom: Blood in Urine

In cases of pediatric bladder cancer, the ratio of benign to malignant is usually much higher for ages 0-13 than for patients 13-19. Even teens will have over a 90% chance of having only benign causes of hematuria, including, but not limited to, stones, trauma, etc.

Only a small percentage of children who may complain of blood in their urine will actually have bladder cancer. However, the presence of blood in the urine is the body's way of signaling that a problem exists, and for that reason, the primary job of the pediatric caregiver is to rule it out completely as a cause of the bleeding. In addition, while unusual, it is worth noting that bladder cancer can still occur in children who have in utero carcinogenic exposure.

Blood in urine The primary symptom in most children is blood in the urine, which will appear bright red or orange. If the child is well-hydrated, it may appear pink. Blood may be present regardless of pain or burning while urinating, and there may be no other problems with any actual tissues of the urinary system. Just as with adults who discover blood in their urine, this is always a concerning finding and should not be ignored.

4. Diagnostic Procedures

A biopsy may be performed to obtain small pieces of tissue from the mass. The tissue will then be examined in a pathology laboratory. For bladder masses in adults, transurethral resection (TUR) is often the standard of care. However, the diagnosis of bladder cancer in children cannot be made by the surgical urologists using TUR alone. TUR can be a part of a staging procedure, but it must be followed by a teaching facility pathologist review of the slides. Pediatric tumors tend to be on or near the surface so a transurethral biopsy is less helpful. Biopsy does have a risk of spreading the tumor through the body and must be undertaken with caution. More commonly, if biopsy is needed in a child with a known or suspected pediatric cancer, it would be done during an operation in an operating room under general anesthesia. Biopsy provides microscopic structure of the cells by a skilled pathologist. Biopsy results are an important part of treatment decisions.

Imaging studies are essential for initially finding and localizing a tumor. Ultrasound uses sound waves to create an image of internal tissues. This test may be improved through using a special ultrasound that is placed in the body to visualize blood vessels and other tissues. Blood tests may also be performed prior to anesthesia to measure kidney function and complete blood counts. If a mass in the bladder is present (most likely a rhabdomyosarcoma in a child less than 10 years old), an MRI may be sufficient for diagnosis, particularly if an advanced MRI was performed before any biopsy as well as have imaging done on the day of or before the biopsy. Appropriate advanced MRI sequences must be used to assist with diagnosis if imaging has not already been performed at a facility familiar with performing imaging tests on pediatric patients (i.e. a pediatric cancer center with a member hospital of the Children's Oncology Group). Ideally, this advanced imaging would be performed before any biopsy.

4.1. Imaging Studies and Biopsy

• Biopsy - No single test can diagnose bladder cancer. Samples are taken from the tumor (biopsy) and are examined under a microscope to determine the type of cancer. Before the biopsy, the patient is given anesthesia and pain medication. The patient may feel some pressure but the procedure is usually not painful. The inside of the body is visualized with a cystoscope, and then the cystoscopic biopsy device is inserted through the cystoscope in order to take a sample of the bladder. The physician uses a cystoscope to look inside the bladder and remove a small piece of tissue for examination. The biopsy sample is evaluated by a pathologist, who will make a final diagnosis and may perform a number of additional tests of the tissue biopsy, such as DNA tests. A biopsy of the mass is the only way to make a definite diagnosis of bladder cancer, and imaging studies will help delineate the areas that the biopsy needs to cover.

• Imaging Studies - Since ultrasonography is usually the first study physicians choose, almost all children with bladder masses will undergo this test. Ultrasonography, a technique based on the reflection of ultrasound waves at tissue interfaces, is the most widely used method to evaluate bladder masses due to its wide availability, relatively low cost, lack of ionizing radiation, and good resolution of the bladder wall layers. MRI and CT are recommended because they can provide information about the extent of disease and detect metastases, both of which are important for treatment and prognosis. These studies are generally performed without contrast and it is reported that a CT scan with contrast accumulates in the reparatum in tumors at specific sites, which can be a helpful finding for diagnosing bladder cancer. The standard of care for diagnosing bladder cancer is MRI or CT (with contrast) and this is the strategy that will often be recommended by your child's physician.

5. Staging and Grading of Pediatric Bladder Cancer

It is generally agreed that there is a significant proportion of tumors in young patients that are of a high clinical stage and high grade. This observation is different from renal cancer in children where most renal tumors in children are diagnosed at an early stage and with a relatively good prognosis compared to the RCC cases in adults. Staging of pelvic malignancies, also bladder cancer, is performed with direct diagnostic methods such as cystoscopy with biopsy and with pelvic imaging methods, at present computer tomography (CT) and magnetic resonance imaging (MRI). One of the widely used staging methods of urinary bladder cancer is based on the TNM classification system, which assesses the depth of infiltration by the primary tumor (T stage), involvement of lymph nodes by metastatic spread (N stage), and the presence/absence of tumor metastases in distant organs (M stage). To assess the depth of local tumor infiltration within the bladder wall (T stage), tumor biopsies of the bladder wall are usually performed during the initial cystoscopy. In the group of primary bladder cancer patients, however, systemic preoperative instrumental and imaging examinations might also be important to assess the degree of tumor biologically and molecularly estimated intra-vesical infiltration, distant tumor spread, and distant lymph nodes (LN) involvement.

There is a general agreement that bladder cancer presents as a more advanced stage in younger patients than in the older ones. In a review by Fernandez et al., it was reported that muscle-invasive disease is three times more common in children and adolescents than in individuals over 20 years of age. Therefore, pediatric bladder cancer is more frequently classified as muscle-invasive at diagnosis. Diagnosis of bladder cancer in children should be based on histological examination of biopsied material. According to the 2016 WHO classification, tumors should be graded as urothelial papilloma (low grade), papillary urothelial neoplasm of low malignant potential (PUNLMP), low-grade Ta carcinoma, low-grade T1 carcinoma, high-grade Ta carcinoma, high-grade T1 carcinoma, high-grade carcinoma in situ, micropapillary and micropapillary variant urothelial carcinoma, nested carcinoma, clear cell adenocarcinoma, and high-grade urothelial carcinoma.

5.1. TNM Classification System

While technical and logistic difficulties in tumor, node, and metastasis (TNM) staging do exist in children, encompassing changes in anatomy, physiology, and histopathologic markers, the TNM classification is recommended by the International Society of Pediatric Oncology, the Children's Oncology Group, and the Society of Pediatric Radiology. Even with numerous differences between the heterogeneous nature of pediatric and adult cancers, some guidelines suggest the use of the adult TNM when classifying pediatric GU malignancies. Squamous cell carcinoma and adenocarcinoma of pediatric urogenital system, while often associated with somatic genetic alterations commonly found in adult tumors, have differences in significantly mutated genes, affected pathways and gene fusions related to development. Additionally, differing environments, costimulatory and immune escape pathways, and the extent and urgency of therapy may contribute to differences in disease behavior and progression.

The TNM classification system, developed by the Union for International Cancer Control and the American Joint Committee on Cancer, is favored for stage and grade classification of pediatric bladder malignancies. Despite the well-known differences in pediatric and adult bladder cancer, this classification system remains an important and valid tool for planning therapy and for analyzing prognosis and outcome. Explicit data guiding adjustments for pediatric cases is lacking, although modifications for staging rhabdomyosarcoma of the genitourinary tract and selecting treatment based on this modified staging have been proposed. Rhabdomyosarcoma is staged on Spiegel criteria, and outcomes vary significantly depending on stage. In order to account for variations in outcomes, diminish confounding factors, and choose optimal therapeutic options, many trials have selectively utilized Omang criteria, which divides stage III into subgroups based on more accurate information.

Tnm classification system favored for pediatric bladder cancer staging.

6. Treatment Modalities

Cystoscopic resection of bladder tumors and transurethral resection (TURB) are essential for histological diagnosis and staging. Mostly, pediatric BC needs more radical surgery, either partial or radical cystectomy. In adults, if hydrodistension of the bladder does not help in the detection or diagnosis of a bladder lesion, hyperhydration during the diagnostic cystoscopy is recommended. For a definitive diagnosis, MRI with or without contrast is necessary. MRI can help with staging and to look for muscle-invasive disease. CT scan of the chest and an X-ray can show evidence of pulmonary metastasis. Chemotherapy and radiotherapy will be employed only once the involved tissues become tumorous.

To date, no defined stratification applies in managing pediatric BC given its rarity. There are no uniform treatment guidelines in managing the disease due to the lack of prospective randomized data and low bx numbers with different clinical presentations encompassing a broad range of staging and grading. This limitation leaves evidence in managing this patient population on experience and extrapolated data from adult BC. When planning treatment in children, the most common advice is to adhere to the bladder cancer guidelines used for standard adult care. However, it has been suggested that regardless of the chosen therapeutic algorithm and the treatment response, all children with BC should be managed in a tertiary pediatric or adult center with full urological and oncological capabilities. It was stated that children had more muscle-invasive and advanced staged disease at diagnosis but a favorable prognosis. A recent multicenter review by Paner et al. summarized that treatment modalities for pediatric BC are divided into three: surgery, chemotherapy, and radiation therapy.

6.1. Surgery, Chemotherapy, and Radiation Therapy

Radiotherapy is currently rarely used in pediatric bladder cancer. This is for a variety of reasons including concerns about prostate exposure to the youngest children, the difficulty of collecting and retaining a full bladder to minimize irradiation to adjacent tissues, and patients' ability to lie still for a long time requiring radiation therapy. However, radiotherapy can be used as part of a palliative care plan. Tumor necrosis is the expected outcome, rather than a cure. An example of the use of radiotherapy can be found in a patient requiring rapid tumor debulking before stoma formation to help with symptoms associated with bladder outlet obstruction due to a huge tumor burden.

The chemotherapy regime generally used is ifosfamide, mixed daily for 5 days with etoposide, every 21 days for 3 courses. Other chemotherapy treatment regimens have emerged and include regimens with carboplatin, cisplatin, or doxorubicin, some of which are used as single drugs or combinations. Radiation Therapy

Transurethral Resection of Tumor (TURBT): The first-line treatment for patients with NMI UC is TURBT. Response to chemotherapy is often optimal following complete TURBT, therefore it is preferred to perform TURBT first and later re-resect the tumor base. Radical Cystectomy: Radical cystectomy is necessary when a bladder tumor invades the bladder muscle. Previously, radical cystectomy was performed after neoadjuvant chemotherapy and subsequent induction chemotherapy. The rationale for giving both neoadjuvant and adjuvant chemotherapy stems from the evidence in adults for this method. Chemotherapy

Surgery

7. Prognosis and Survival Rates

Prognosis is always a "work-in-progress" as new integrating factors are always considered as treatment improves. Some bladder cancer tumors have genes or molecular changes that are likely to mean a worse prognosis, and testing your child's cancer may not be useful in the coming years. These advances are known as molecular pathology or gene-expression studies.

Survival rate: It is difficult for your child's doctor to assess a true survival rate without definitive knowledge about a tumor's stage, grade, and other factors. As much as we can generalize, for kidney and bladder tumors that have not spread beyond the blood vessels, the five-year survival rate can be as high as 85%. Survival rates for older patients are slightly lower than that for younger people. If the tumor has spread outside the kidney or bladder, the prognosis is significantly worse. For those with the more advanced disease, overall survival rates can be up to 20-50%. However, remember that every patient is different and can be expected to have different outcomes. Some bladder tumors have spread before they are diagnosed and have a worse prognosis. In addition, patients who experience local symptoms (such as pain, unable to urinate, or blood in their urine) are far more likely to experience generalized symptoms such as weight loss, fever, etc.

Prognostic factors: Other factors of importance include the presence of symptoms, the number of other tumors, and the symptoms. In addition, the grade can indicate the likelihood of spreading to nearby tissues and the aggressiveness of a tumor. The grade is usually determined by a pathologist looking at the tissue under the microscope.

Stage: The extent of the tumor at the time of biopsy is also an important factor. It is important that the biopsy tissue be taken from the entire tumor so that we know the stage and other attributes of the tumor. There are different staging systems for bladder tumors. Survival rate cannot be predicted without knowing the stage of the tumor.

Age at diagnosis: The prognosis of pediatric bladder tumors is associated with the age at which the tumor is diagnosed. The younger the patient, the better the prognosis.

What is the prognosis? The prognosis for children with bladder tumors is determined by a variety of predictors or prognostic factors. These prognostic factors are used to create treatment guidelines or standards because they have a direct impact on cure. It is important to discuss all of these factors with your child's doctor.

Prognosis and survival rates

7.1. Positive Outlook for Kids After Treatment

Children treated for cancer are encouraged to return to normal activities as they are able. Children and teens who have been treated for bladder cancer might have some things in their medical records that give them problems later in life. For example, certain cancer treatments can result in problems with fertility, so teens who are treated for bladder cancer may want to withhold some of their sperm or eggs before treatment. And some treatment might cause health issues that don't show up until years later, when they may be mistaken for something else. To help doctors monitor a child's health after cancer treatment, it's important for them to record the name of the cancer and the type of treatment they received, as well as the doctors they saw and when they saw them. It's also helpful to keep an eye on medical records beyond cancer: children should keep records of their medical history in a central file, and their family doctor should keep a list of treatments and tests they've had.

The outlook is good for kids treated successfully for bladder cancer. Most will continue regular checkups with the doctors for years to come. Kids being checked for bladder cancer need to see a specialist. A pediatric oncologist treats children and teens with cancer. Other childhood cancer specialists focus on surgery, radiation, and more. After treatment, some kids might work with a specialist called a urologist who focuses on the urinary system. Experts called pediatric care (palliative) specialists help kids with cancer, too. Palliative care specialists are experts in dealing with pain, ranging from pain medications to massage therapy. Many hospitals have programs for children with cancer and their families that include doctors, nurses, pharmacists, social workers, child life specialists, nutritionists, and others who can explain the disease, guide treatment, and support the whole family.